AGELESS BEAUTY
"Nurturing Your Skin Inside and Out"

Mamie C. Fenner

2

Brand ©(**2024**) by(**Mamie C. Fenner**)

3

CHAPTER 1

Understanding Ageless: Beauty

Defining timeless beauty beyond physicalAppearance:
Timeless beauty is further than skin-deep. It's about nurturing your skin while embracing the wisdom of experience. It involves a holistic approach, balancing skincare, nutrition, and life. A healthy diet, an acclimatized skincare routine, stress operation, exercise, and tone- acceptance

all play pivotal places. It's not just about looking immature but feeling confident and embracing every stage of life with grace. timeless beauty is the harmony between minding for your body, mind, and spirit, creating a dateless gleam that radiates from within.

Exploring the cerebral and emotional aspects of beauty:

 Beauty is not just about looks — it's about how it makes us feel. When we see a beautiful commodity, like an evening or a smiling face, it frequently makes us feel good outside. It can make us happy, impressed, or inspired. Our passions about beauty can affect how we see ourselves and others.

Occasionally, people who are allowed as seductive might be seen as further confident or friendly. This can impact how we interact with them. But beauty is different for everyone. What one person finds beautiful might not be the same for someone differently. That is because beauty is shaped by what we learn from our culture, society, and particular guests.

Feeling beautiful or not feeling beautiful can affect how we feel about ourselves. Sometimes, we might compare ourselves to what we suppose is" beautiful" and feel like we do not measure up. But it's important to flash back that beauty comes in numerous forms, and accepting ourselves and others for who we're is really important.

Understanding the emotional and cerebral corridor of beauty means knowing how it affects how we suppose and feel. It's about accepting that beauty is further than just appearances ,it's about feeling good about ourselves and appreciating the oneness and differences in everyone.

Preface to the holistic approach to skincare and heartiness:

Holistic skincare and heartiness go beyond face-position treatments; they encompass a complete approach that considers the interconnectedness of our body, mind, and spirit. Rather than fastening solely on external symptoms or beauty enterprises, the holistic approach acknowledges the significance of nurturing overall well- being to achieve vibrant and healthy skin.

This approach recognizes that our skin reflects our internal health and is informed by colorful factors, including life, feelings, nutrition, and terrain. By integrating practices that promote balance and harmony within the body, mind, and spirit, holistic skincare seeks to address the root causes of skin issues while enhancing overall health.

Embracing holistic skincare involves espousing an aware life that includes nourishing the body with proper nutrition, staying doused , managing stress, getting quality sleep, regular exercise, and using natural products that support skin health. It emphasizes the significance of tone- care, tone- acceptance, and awareness practices to foster inner balance and radiate external beauty.

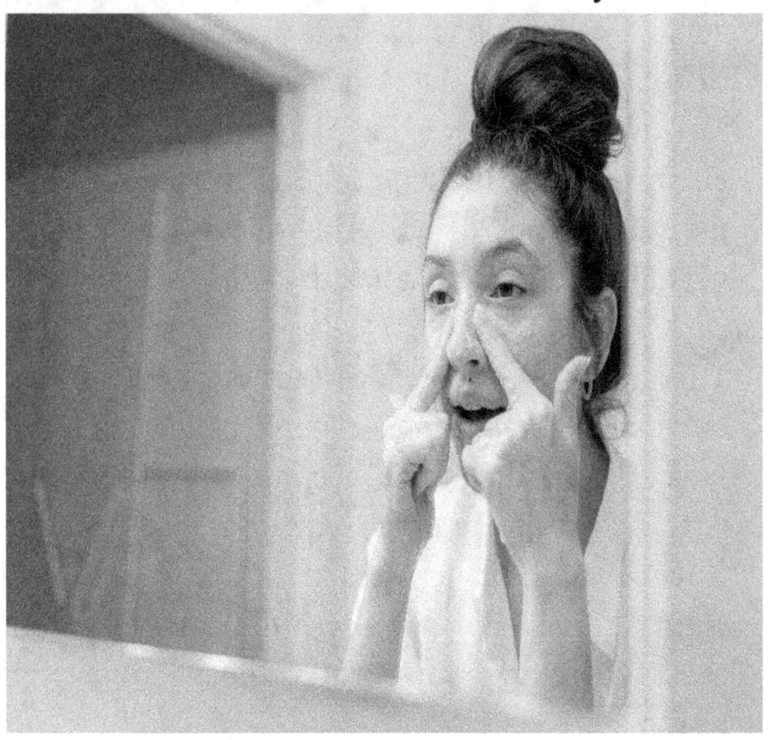

In substance, the holistic approach to skincare and heartiness is about treating the body as a whole, feting the community between internal well- being and external beauty. By prioritizing a harmonious life and embracing practices that promote overall health, holistic skincare aims to produce a foundation for radiant skin and a more fulfilling, balanced life.

Chapter 2

Inner Aliment for Timeless Beauty:

True beauty frequently starts from within, reflecting the aliment we give to our bodies through our salutary choices. Inner aliment for dateless beauty involves consuming foods rich in essential nutrients that not only support overall health but also contribute to radiant skin, helping maintain an immature gleam and vitality.

The connection between diet, nutrition, and skin health:

The relationship between diet, nutrition, and skin health is intricate, as what we eat significantly influences the appearance, texture, and overall condition of your skin.

A diet abundant in fruits, vegetables, whole grains, lean proteins, and healthy fats offers a spectrum of vitamins, antioxidants, and minerals crucial for skin health. For instance

- **Antioxidant-rich Foods:** Berries, citrus fruits, leafy greens, and nuts contain antioxidants that combat free radicals, reducing skin damage and supporting a youthful appearance.

- **Omega-3 Fatty Acids:** Found in fatty fish, flaxseeds, and walnuts, omega-3s help maintain skin elasticity, hydration, and overall suppleness.

- **Vitamin C Sources:** Foods like oranges, strawberries, and bell peppers are high in vitamin C, aiding collagen production and promoting skin firmness.

- **Vitamin E Enriched Foods:** Almonds, spinach, and avocados contain vitamin E, which protects skin from oxidative stress and supports skin health.

- **Hydration:** Drinking ample water and consuming hydrating foods like watermelon, cucumber, and celery keeps the skin hydrated, maintaining its elasticity and a healthy appearance.

Remember, while focusing on external skin care is important, the benefits truly amplify when combined with a diet rich in nutrients that support skin health from the inside out. Inner nourishment not only contributes to a radiant complexion but also supports overall well-being, reflecting timeless beauty that emanates from a well-nourished body.

- **Collagen Production:** Collagen, a protein crucial for skin elasticity and firmness, is influenced by dietary components. Foods rich in vitamin C, such as citrus fruits,

strawberries, and broccoli, aid collagen synthesis, contributing to skin strength and suppleness.

- **Omega-3 Fatty Acids:** Consumption of omega-3 fatty acids found in fatty fish like salmon, chia seeds, and walnuts helps maintain skin integrity. These fatty acids support the skin's lipid barrier, improving moisture retention and reducing inflammation, thereby enhancing skin texture and reducing dryness

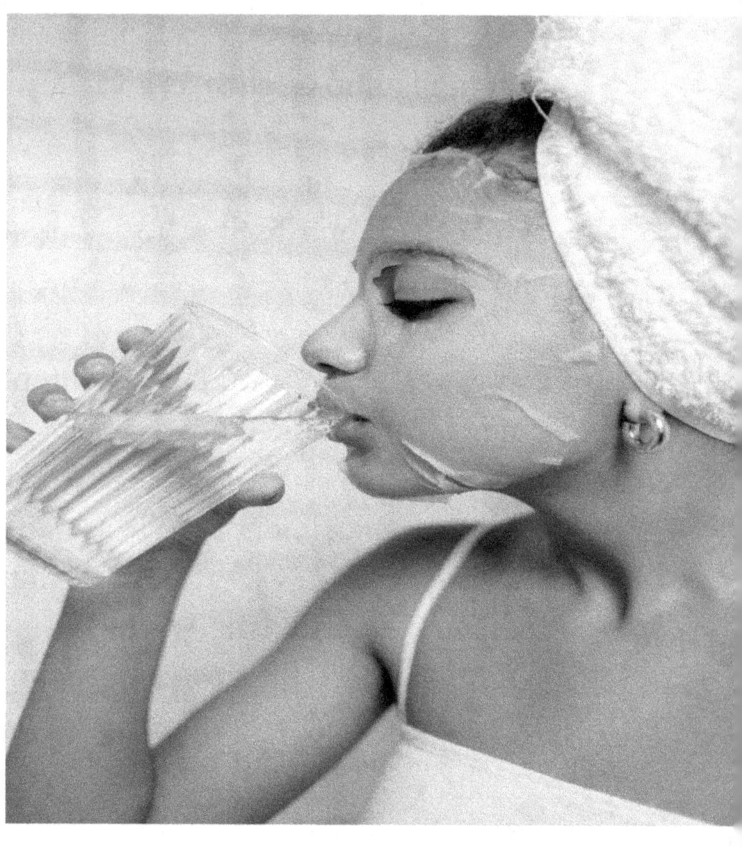

- **Antioxidants Combatting Free Radicals:** Vitamins A, C, and E, as well as other antioxidants found in colorful fruits and vegetables like carrots, berries, and spinach, help neutralize free radicals.

These compounds protect the skin from oxidative stress caused by UV rays and environmental pollutants, thus minimizing premature aging signs like wrinkles and fine lines.

- **Hydration and Water Content:** Proper hydration achieved through water input and consumption of hydrating foods like cucumbers, tomatoes, and watermelon is vital for skin health. Hydration helps maintain skin humidity, precluding blankness and promoting a rotund and immature appearance.

- **Inflammatory Foods Impacting Skin:** Some studies suggest that high- glycemic-indicator foods, similar as reused carbohydrates and sugars, might complicate acne and skin inflammation. Again, a diet rich in whole grains, fruits, and vegetables helps maintain stable blood sugar situations and potentially reduces skin issues.

- **Probiotics and Gut Health:** Probiotic-rich foods like yogurt, kefir, and fermented vegetables support gut health. A healthy gut microbiome may appreciatively impact skin conditions like acne and eczema by reducing inflammation and perfecting skin hedge function.

In summary, a well- rounded and balanced diet conforming to nutrient- thick foods plays a vital part in nurturing healthy and radiant skin. Understanding the relationship between diet, nutrition, and skin health empowers individualities to make informed salutary choices that support optimal skin function and appearance.

Pressing foods that promote immature skin:

Several foods are known for their capability to promote immature skin by furnishing essential nutrients and antioxidants. These are some exemplifications.:

- **Berries:** Blueberries, strawberries, snorts, and blackberries are rich in antioxidants like vitamin C and anthocyanins. These composites combat oxidative stress, reducing damage from free revolutionaries and contributing to an immature complexion.

- **Adipose Fish:** Salmon, mackerel, and sardines are high in omega- 3 adipose acids. These adipose acids help maintain skin hydration, pliantness, and reduce inflammation, keeping the skin supple and immature.

- **Nuts and Seeds:** Almonds, walnuts, chia seeds, and flaxseeds are sources of omega- 3s, vitamin E, and antioxidants. They cover against free revolutionaries, support collagen products, and help maintain skin pliantness.

- **Avocado:** Rich in healthy fats, vitamins E and C, and antioxidants, avocados aid in skin hydration, protection against UV damage, and promote collagen conflation for establishment, immature skin

.

- **lush Flora:** Spinach, kale, and other lush flora give vitamins A, C, and K along with antioxidants. They help repair and renew skin cells, fight inflammation, and contribute to a radiant complexion.

- **Orange and Yellow Fruits/Vegetables:** Carrots, sweet potatoes, bell peppers, and oranges are loaded with beta- carotene, which converts to vitaminA. Vitamin A helps maintain skin health, form apkins, and promote skin cell development for a fresh appearance.

- **Tomatoes:** Rich in lycopene, tomatoes cover the skin from sun damage and ameliorate skin texture. They act as a natural sunscreen, reducing the dangerous goods of UV radiation on the skin.

- **Green Tea:** This libation contains polyphenols that have potent antioxidant and anti-inflammatory parcels. Regular consumption may help cover the skin from damage and maintain an immature appearance.

Including these foods in a balanced diet can help nourish the skin from within, furnishing essential nutrients and antioxidants that support an immature and radiant complexion.

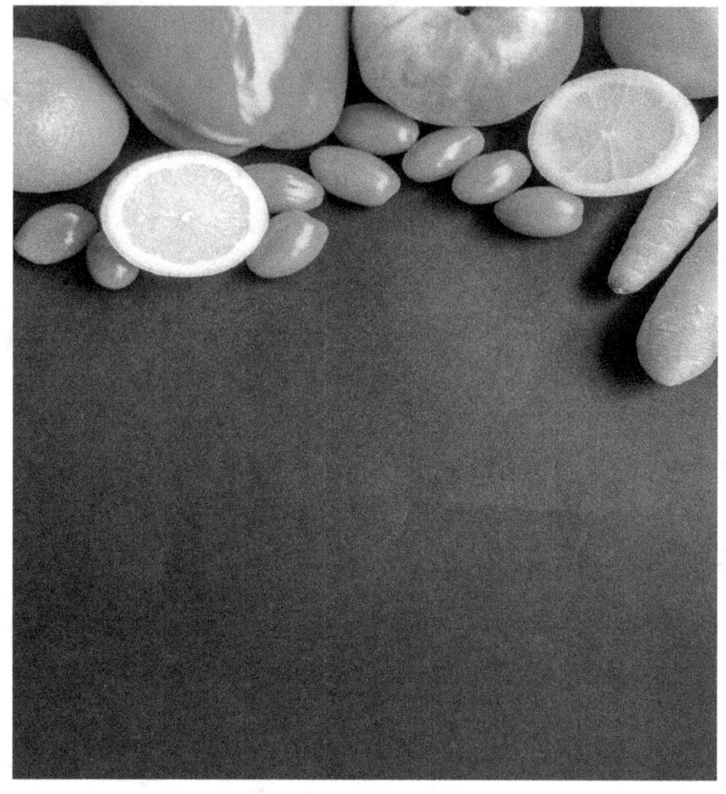

Tips on creating a balanced, skin- nourishing diet and hydration practices:

Creating a balanced, skin- nourishing diet and maintaining proper hydration are essential for promoting healthy and glowing skin. Here are some tips to achieve this

Balanced Diet for Skin Health:
Include a Variety of Nutrient-thick Foods Incorporate a different range of fruits, vegetables, whole grains, spare proteins(similar as fish, flesh, tofu), healthy fats(like avocados, nuts, seeds), and legumes. These give essential vitamins, minerals, antioxidants, and omega- 3 adipose acids salutary for skin health.

Prioritize Antioxidant- Rich Foods:
Berries, lush flora, citrus fruits, and various vegetables are rich in antioxidants. These combat free revolutionaries, cover against UV damage, and contribute to an immature complexion.

Healthy Fats for Skin Ailment:
Omega- 3 adipose acids set up in adipose fish, flaxseeds, and walnuts support skin hydration, reduce inflammation, and maintain skin pliantness.

conclude for Foods Supporting Collagen product Include foods rich in vitamin C (oranges, strawberries, bell peppers) and amino acids(spare flesh, dairy, legumes) to support collagen conflation for establishment and supple skin.

Stay Doused:
Hydrate from within by drinking plenty of water throughout the day. Herbal teas, coconut water, and invested water with fruits or cucumber are also excellent hydration choices.

Hydration Practices for Skin Health:

Regular Water Intake: Aim for at least 8-10 cups (64-80 ounces) of water daily, adjusting based on climate, activity level, and individual needs.

Consistent Hydration Throughout the Day: Sip water consistently rather than consuming large amounts infrequently. Carry a reusable water bottle to ensure regular intake.

Monitor Urine Color: Keep an eye on urine color; ideally, it should be pale yellow, indicating proper hydration.

Moisturize Externally: Use a suitable moisturizer to support skin hydration externally, especially after bathing or washing your face to lock in moisture.

Limit Dehydrating Beverages: Minimize consumption of dehydrating drinks like alcohol, excessive caffeine, and sugary beverages that can contribute to dehydration.

By adopting a diet rich in essential nutrients and maintaining proper hydration practices, you can nourish your skin from within, supporting its health and achieving a radiant complexion.

Skincare Regimens for Ageless Radiance:

Creating a skincare regimen focused on ageless radiance involves a comprehensive approach that addresses specific skin concerns while promoting overall skin health and vitality. Here's a suggested skincare routine:

Morning Skincare Routine:

Cleansing: Begin with a gentle cleanser suited for your skin type to remove overnight impurities and excess oil.

Toning: Use a toner to rebalance the skin's pH levels and prep it for better absorption of subsequent products.

Serum Application: Apply a serum containing antioxidants like vitamin C or hyaluronic acid to combat free radicals, promote collagen production, and hydrate the skin.

Eye Cream: Use an eye cream targeting concerns like puffiness, dark circles, or fine lines around the eyes.

Moisturizing: Apply a lightweight, hydrating moisturizer with SPF to protect against UV damage. Sunscreen is crucial, even on cloudy days, to prevent premature aging.

Night time Skincare Regimen:
Makeup junking/ scrubbing To get relief of makeup, dirt, and adulterants that have accumulated throughout the day, use a mild makeup way and also give your skin a thorough scrubbing.

Exfoliation(1-2 times per week): slip to get relieve of dead skin cells, which will stimulate cell development and make your skin look further radiant. select a mild exfoliant grounded on the kind of skin on your body.

Toning: After sanctifying or slipping, use a color to restore equilibrium to the skin.

Treatment Products: To address particular issues like fine lines, wrinkles, or uneven skin tone, apply technical treatments like retinoids or peptides.

Hydration: To seal in humidity and restore damaged skin as you sleep, use a nutritional night cream or face oil painting as a finishing touch.

Extra Advice

The secret is to be harmonious: follow your skincare authority religiously to start seeing benefits over time.

Customize to Your Needs: Tailor your regimen based on your skin type, concerns, and preferences. Consult a dermatologist for personalized advice if needed.

Stay Hydrated and Eat Well: Maintain a healthy diet and stay hydrated for overall skin health.

Protect from Sun Exposure: Use sunscreen daily and avoid prolonged sun exposure to prevent premature aging and protect against UV damage.

Remember, while a skincare routine can significantly contribute to ageless radiance, a holistic approach encompassing lifestyle factors, nutrition, hydration, and stress management is equally crucial for maintaining youthful and radiant skin.

Chapter 3

Effective skincare routines for different ages and skin types

Certainly, skincare routines should be adapted based on both age and skin type to address specific concerns and support overall skin health. Here are suggested skincare routines for different ages and skin types:

Skincare Routine for Teens (Ages 13-19):

Cleansing: Use a gentle cleanser twice daily to remove excess oil, dirt, and impurities without stripping the skin.

- **Moisturizing:** Apply a lightweight, oil-free moisturizer to hydrate without clogging pores.

- **Sun Protection:** Use a broad-spectrum sunscreen daily to protect from UV damage and prevent future skin issues.

- **Spot Treatment:** Use targeted spot treatments with ingredients like benzoyl peroxide or salicylic acid for acne breakouts, if necessary.

Skincare Routine for 20s and 30s:

- **Cleansing:** Cleanse twice daily using a gentle cleanser suitable for your skin type.

- **Exfoliation:** Include exfoliation (1-2 times a week) to promote cell turnover and maintain a bright complexion.

- **Serums:** Apply serums containing antioxidants, hyaluronic acid, or vitamin C to address specific concerns like hydration, brightening, or early signs of aging.

- **Moisturizing:** Use a lightweight moisturizer in the morning and a more nourishing one at night.

- **Sunscreen:** Daily use of SPF is crucial to prevent premature aging and protect against sun damage.

- **Eye Cream:** Start incorporating an eye cream to address early signs of aging around the eyes.

Skincare Routine for 40s and Beyond:

- **Gentle Cleansing:** Use a gentle cleanser to avoid stripping the skin of essential oils, which can become drier with age.

- **Antioxidant Serums:** Apply serums containing potent antioxidants, peptides, and retinoids to target fine lines, wrinkles, and age spots.

- **Hydration and Moisturizing:** Use richer, deeply hydrating moisturizers to combat dryness and maintain skin elasticity.

- **Eye Creams and Treatments:** Use specialized eye creams and treatments for more targeted care around the delicate eye area.

- **Sun Protection:** Continue consistent use of sunscreen to prevent further sun damage and signs of aging.

Skincare Routines for Different Skin Types:

- **Dry Skin:** Focus on hydrating products including creamy cleansers, rich moisturizers, and hyaluronic acid-based serums to lock in moisture.

- **Oily/Acne-Prone Skin:** Use gentle, non-comedogenic products and incorporate salicylic acid or benzoyl peroxide to control excess oil and treat acne.

- **Combination Skin:** Balance the routine with products that cater to both oily and dry areas. Use lightweight, oil-free products on the oily zones and hydrating products on drier areas.

- **Sensitive Skin:** Opt for fragrance-free, hypoallergenic products to minimize irritation. Patch test new products and use calming ingredients like aloe vera or chamomile.

Tailoring skincare routines to age and skin type ensures that specific concerns are addressed while promoting overall skin health and vitality. Consulting a dermatologist or skincare professional can provide personalized guidance based on individual needs and concerns.

Recommendations for cleansing, exfoliation, moisturizing, and protection:

Here are recommendations for each step of a skincare routine:

Cleansing:

Cleanser for Different Skin Types:

Dry Skin: CeraVe Hydrating Cleanser or La Roche-Posay Toleriane Hydrating Gentle Cleanser.

Oily

/Acne-Prone Skin: Cetaphil Daily Facial Cleanser or Neutrogena Oil-Free Acne Wash.

Combination

 Skin: Bioderma Sensibio H2O Micellar Water or Paula's Choice RESIST Perfectly Balanced Foaming Cleanser.

Sensitive

 Skin: Aveeno Ultra-Calming Hydrating Gel Cleanser or Vanicream Gentle Facial Cleanser.

EXFOLIATION:

Exfoliants for Different Needs:

Chemical Exfoliants: Paula's Choice Skin Perfecting 2% BHA Liquid Exfoliant or The Ordinary Glycolic Acid 7% Toning Solution.

Physical

Exfoliants (for sensitive skin, use sparingly): Dermalogica Daily Microfoliant or First Aid Beauty Facial Radiance Pads.

Moisturizing:

Moisturizers for Various Skin Types:

Dry Skin: CeraVe Moisturizing Cream or Eucerin Advanced Repair Cream.

- **Oily**

/Acne-Prone Skin: Neutrogena Hydro Boost Water Gel or La Roche-Posay Effaclar Mat Moisturizer.

- **Combination**
- **Skin:** Drunk Elephant Protini Cream or Belif The True Cream Aqua Bomb.
- **Sensitive Skin:** Cetaphil Daily Hydrating Lotion or Vanicream Moisturizing Cream.

SUN PROTECTION

Sunscreen Recommendations:
EltaMD UV Clear Broad-Spectrum SPF 46 or La Roche-Posay Anthelios Melt-in Milk Sunscreen SPF 100 for face.Neutrogena Ultra Sheer Dry-Touch Sunscreen SPF 50 or Supergoop! Everyday Sunscreen SPF 50 for body.

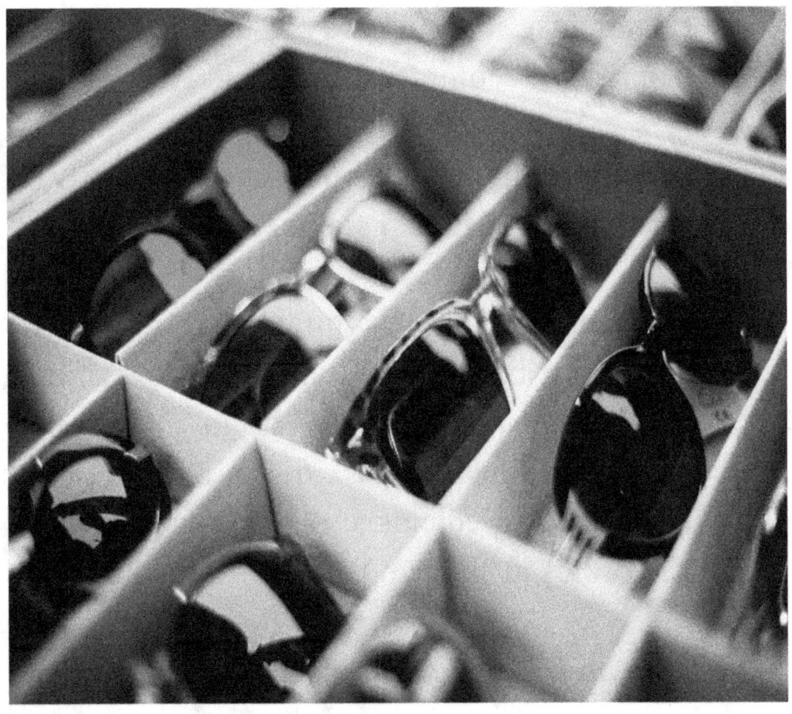

Remember, these recommendations can serve as a starting point, but it's essential to consider your skin's individual needs, sensitivities, and reactions to products. Patch-testing new products and gradually introducing them into your routine helps to ensure they work well with your skin. Additionally, consistency is key in seeing results with any skincare routine. If you have specific concerns or persistent issues, consulting a dermatologist is always advisable for personalized recommendations and guidance.

Understanding the importance of natural ingredients and their role in skincare:

Understanding the significance of natural ingredients in skincare involves recognizing their beneficial properties and how they contribute to healthier skin. Here are reasons why natural ingredients are valued and examples of their roles in skincare:

Gentle and Safe Formulations:

Aloe Vera: Known for its soothing and hydrating properties, it calms irritated skin and aids in healing.Chamomile: Anti-inflammatory and calming, ideal for sensitive or irritated skin.

Nourishment and Hydration:

Hyaluronic Acid: Naturally occurring in the skin, it retains moisture, plumping and hydrating the skin.Jojoba Oil: Mimics the skin's natural oils, moisturizing without clogging pores.

Antioxidant Protection:

Vitamin E: Shields against free radicals, helping to prevent premature aging.Green Tea Extract: Rich in antioxidants, it combats oxidative stress, promoting youthful skin.

Exfoliation and Renewal:

Fruit Enzymes (Pineapple, Papaya): Natural exfoliants that gently remove dead skin cells for a brighter complexion.Sugar or Rice Bran: Provides mild physical exfoliation without causing micro-tears.

Anti-Aging and Collagen Production:

Vitamin C: Fights signs of aging, boosts collagen product, and brightens the skin.Rosehip Seed oil painting High in vitamin A and essential adipose acids, it aids in skin rejuvenation and reduces fine lines.

Antibacterial and Acne- Fighting parcels Tea Tree Oil:

Has antimicrobial parcels, effective in treating acne and blemishes. Honey Natural antibacterial and soothing parcels, salutary for acne-prone skin.

Natural constituents frequently contain smaller synthetic chemicals, reducing the liability of skin vexation or antipathetic responses. They work synergistically with the skin's natural processes, offering a gentle yet effective approach to skincare. Still, it's essential to note that not all natural constituents are suitable for every skin type, and individual perceptivity may vary. Always patch- test new products and consult with a dermatologist if you have specific skin enterprises or disinclination. Using natural constituents on your skin

Tea Tree Oil:

operation: Adulterate tea tree oil painting with a carrier oil painting(like coconut or jojoba oil painting) and apply sparingly to acne-prone areas as a spot treatment. Avoid using unmixed on the skin, especially if you have sensitive skin.

Green Tea:

operation: Pop green tea and let it cool. Use it as a color by applying it with a cotton pad to refresh the skin, reduce inflammation, and give antioxidants.

Oatmeal:

operation: Make an oatmeal face mask by blending oats into a fine greasepaint and mixing it with water or yogurt. Apply the paste to the skin for 10- 15 twinkles, also wash off. It's soothing and helps with blankness or vexation.

Jojoba Oil:

> **Operation:** Apply many drops to damp skin after sanctification as a natural moisturizer. It nearly resembles the skin's natural sebum and is suitable for utmost skin types.

Apple Cider ginger:

> **operation:** Adulterate apple cider ginger with water(1 part ginger to 3- 4 corridor water) and use as a color to balance skin pH. Apply with a cotton pad, leave it for a many twinkles, also wash off or follow with moisturizer.

Rosehip Seed oil:

> **painting operation:** Apply many drops to the face as a moisturizer or add it to your moisturizer. It's rich in antioxidants and suitable for mature or dry skin.

Witch Hazel:

operation: Use witch hazel as a color by applying it to a cotton pad and gently swiping it over the skin. It can help with oiliness and inflammation.

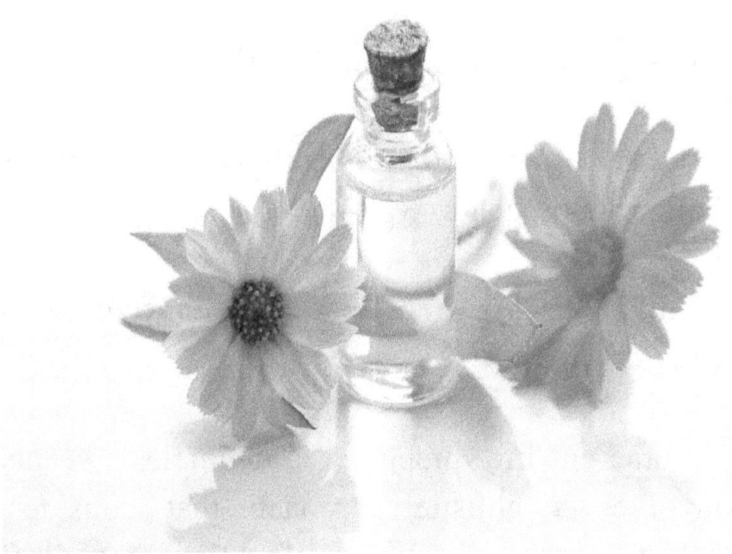

Always perform a patch test before using any natural component to check for implicit antipathetic responses or skin perceptivity. Also, if you have any skin enterprises or conditions, consult a dermatologist before incorporating new constituents into your skincare routine.

Chapter 4

Lifestyle Habits for Timeless Glow:

A dateless gleam frequently comes from a holistic approach to well- being.

Embracing life practices that contribute to timeless beauty:

Embracing life practices for timeless beauty involves a holistic approach that considers colorful aspects of your life. Then are some practices that can contribute to timeless beauty:

Healthy Diet:

Hydration: Drink plenitude of water to keep your skin doused .

Antioxidant-rich Foods: Consume fruits and vegetables high in antioxidants to fight free revolutionaries and promote skin health.

Omega- 3 Adipose Acids: Include foods like salmon, flaxseeds, and walnuts for their anti-inflammatory parcels, serving skin and overall health. Collagen Boosting Foods Incorporate foods like bone broth, berries, and lush flora to support collagen products for skin pliantness.

Skincare Routine:

sanctification: Use a gent cleaner suitable for your skin type.Moisturizing Hydrate your skin with a good moisturizer. Sun Protection Wear sunscreen daily to cover against UV rays.Consistency Stick to a routine that works for your skin and be harmonious.

- **Regular exercise:**

Regular exercise improves blood rotation, leading to healthierskin.Yoga or contemplation can also help reduce stress, which can impact your skin's health.

- **Acceptable Sleep:**

Quality sleep rejuvenates your skin and helps in its form process.

- **Stress operation**:

Practice awareness, contemplation, or pursuits that relax you.Chronic stress can affect skin health, so changing ways to manage stress is pivotal.

- **Avoiding Harmful Habits:**

Smoking Avoid smoking as it accelerates growth and damage skin.Excessive Alcohol Limit alcohol input as it can dehydrate the skin.

- **Regular Skin Checks:**

Pay attention to changes in your skin and seek professional advice if demanded.

- **Positive Outlook and Confidence:**

A positive mindset frequently radiates from within and contributes to an overall gleam.

- **Tone- Care:**

Take time for yourself. Whether it's through skincare routines, cataracts, or pursuits, tone-care is essential.

- **Balance and temperance:**

Strive for balance in all aspects of life, including diet, work, and rest.

- **Consulting Professionals:**

Visit dermatologists or skincare experts for substantiated advice.

Flash back, a dateless gleam is not just about appearance — it's also about feeling good from the inside out. Combining these habits with a positive mindset can help you achieve that radiant, dateless air.

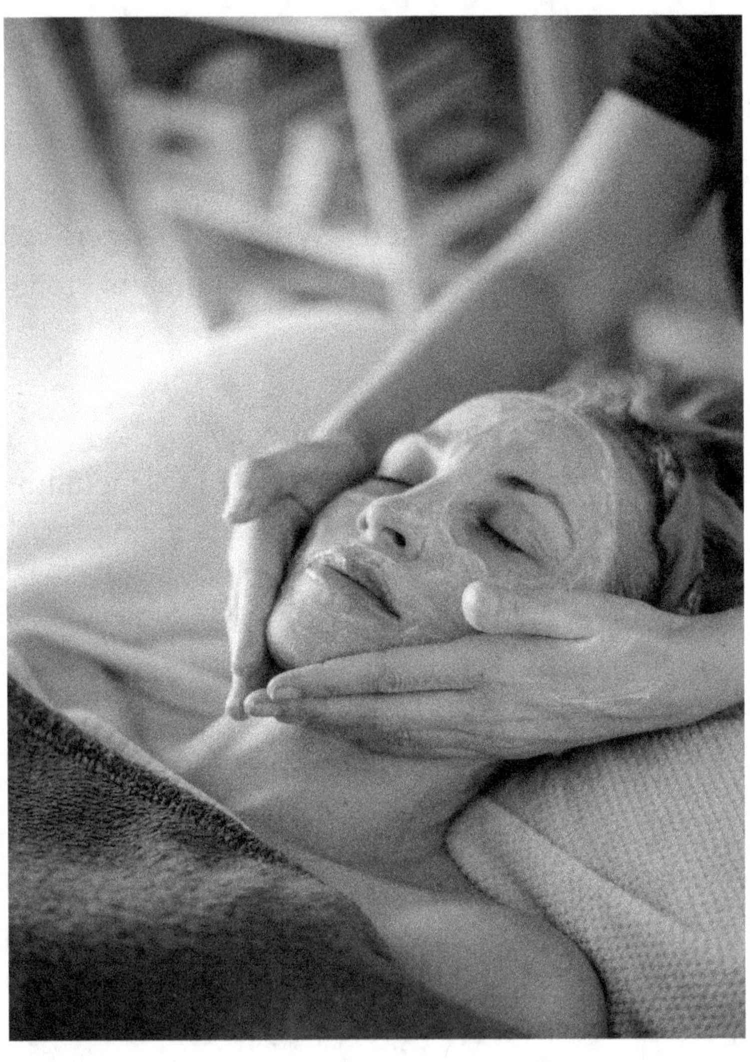

Stress operation ways and their impact on skin health

Stress can significantly impact skin health, often leading to various skin issues such as acne, eczema, psoriasis, rosacea, and premature aging. Managing stress effectively can have a positive impact on skin health. Here are some stress management techniques and how they can benefit your skin:

1. **Mindfulness Meditation:**

Impact on Skin: Reduces inflammation and improves skin conditions aggravated by stress.
How It Helps: By focusing on the present moment, mindfulness meditation reduces cortisol levels, which can alleviate stress-related skin problems.

2. **Deep Breathing Exercises:**

Impact on Skin: Enhances oxygen supply to the skin and reduces stress-induced skin inflammation.

How It Helps: Deep breathing techniques activate the parasympathetic nervous system, promoting relaxation and reducing stress-related skin flare-ups.

3. **Regular Exercise**:

Impact on Skin: Improves blood circulation and helps flush out toxins, leading to a healthier complexion.
How It Helps: Physical activity releases endorphins, reducing stress and promoting better skin health by supplying more oxygen and nutrients to the skin.

4. **Yoga:**

Impact on Skin: Reduces inflammation and promotes relaxation, benefiting skin conditions triggered by stress.
How It Helps: Yoga combines physical movement, controlled breathing, and mindfulness, aiding in stress reduction and improving overall skin health.

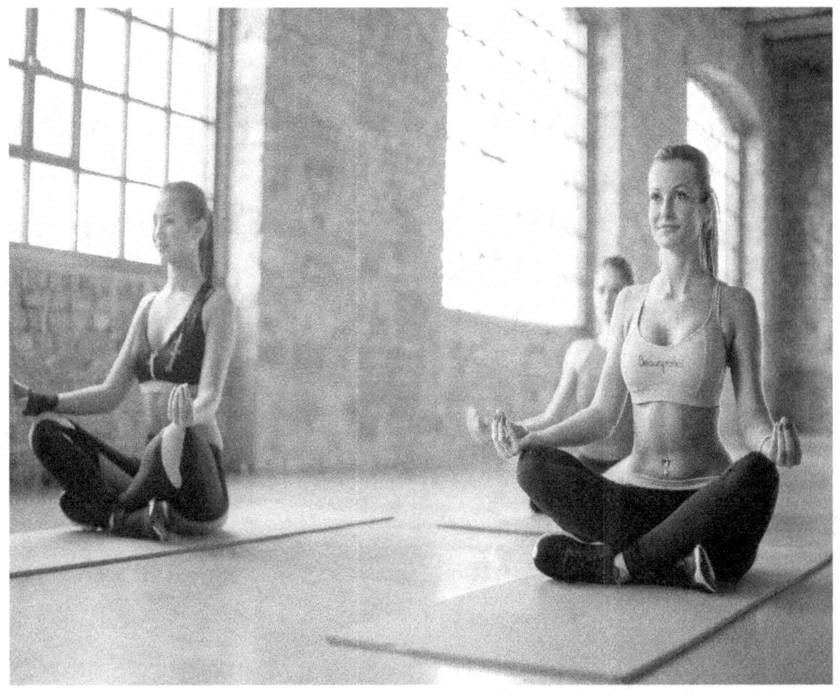

5. Adequate Sleep:

Impact on Skin: Promotes skin repair and regeneration.
How It Helps: Quality sleep allows the skin to repair and rejuvenate, reducing stress-induced skin issues and promoting a healthier complexion.

6. Healthy Eating:

Impact on Skin: Nutrient-rich foods can combat stress-induced skin problems.

How It Helps: Consuming a balanced diet with antioxidants, vitamins, and omega-3 fatty acids supports skin health, counteracting the effects of stress on the skin.

7. Relaxation Techniques:

Impact on Skin: Reduces stress-related skin inflammation and flare-ups.

How It Helps: Engaging in activities such as reading, listening to music, taking baths, or pursuing hobbies relaxes the mind and body, alleviating stress and benefiting skin health.

8. Skincare Rituals as Self-Care:

Impact on Skin: Encourages relaxation and self-care, reducing stress-related skin issues.

How It Helps: Establishing a skincare routine can be a form of self-care that promotes relaxation and reduces stress, contributing to healthier skin.

Managing stress through these techniques not only benefits your mental and physical well-being but also positively impacts your skin health. Incorporating stress management practices into your daily routine can help maintain a healthy and glowing complexion.

Importance of sleep, exercise, and mindfulness in maintaining youthful skin:

Sleep, exercise, and mindfulness play vital roles in maintaining youthful skin by promoting overall health, reducing stress, and supporting skin regeneration. Here's a breakdown of their importance:

1. **Sleep:**

Cellular Repair and Regeneration: During sleep, the body repairs and regenerates tissues, including skin cells. This process helps in maintaining youthful and healthy-looking skin.Collagen Production: Adequate sleep contributes to the production of collagen, which is essential for skin elasticity and preventing wrinkles.Reduced Inflammation: Sufficient sleep reduces inflammation, which can otherwise contribute to skin issues like acne and accelerated aging.

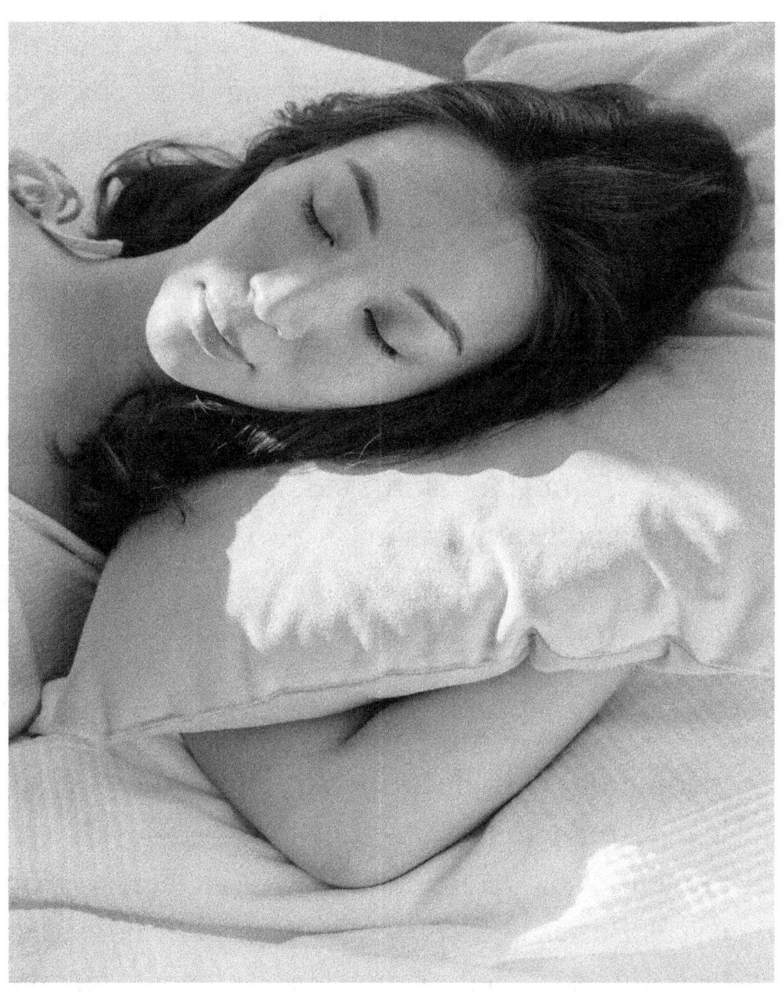

2. **Exercise:**

Improved Blood Circulation: Regular exercise increases blood flow, delivering more oxygen and nutrients to skin cells. This helps in promoting a healthy glow and supports skin health.Stress Reduction: Exercise releases endorphins, reducing stress levels. Lower stress can minimize skin problems exacerbated by stress, such as acne and eczema.Detoxification: Sweating during exercise helps in clearing out toxins from the skin, aiding in maintaining clearer and healthier skin.

3. **Mindfulness**:

Stress Reduction: Mindfulness practices like meditation and deep breathing lower cortisol levels, reducing stress. Lower stress levels can prevent or alleviate stress-related skin issues.Better Sleep Quality: Mindfulness techniques can improve sleep quality, contributing to better skin repair and rejuvenation during sleep.Reduced Inflammation: Mindfulness practices have been linked to lower levels of inflammation, which can benefit overall skin health.

Synergy Among Sleep, Exercise, and Mindfulness:

When combined, these practices create a harmonious effect on the body and skin. Quality sleep enhances the benefits of exercise by aiding in muscle repair and recovery.Mindfulness techniques can complement both sleep and exercise, promoting relaxation and reducing the negative impact of stress on skin health.

Maintaining a balance among adequate sleep, regular exercise, and mindfulness practices contributes not only to youthful skin but also to overall well-being. These lifestyle factors work synergistically to support healthy skin and can help in delaying signs of aging.

Chapter 5:

Embracing Change and Self-Care for Lasting Beauty

Embracing change and practicing self-care are essential elements for lasting beauty that goes beyond physical appearance.

Redefining beauty standards and embracing the aging process:

1. Acceptance of Change:

Mindset Shift: Embrace the natural process of aging as a part of life rather than something to resist. Accepting change with grace can positively impact your perception of beauty.

Adaptability: Embrace changes in your body and appearance, understanding that beauty is not stagnant but evolves over time.

2. Self-Care as a Priority:

Holistic Wellness: Prioritize self-care by attending to physical, mental, and emotional needs.

Healthy Lifestyle: Engage in activities that nourish your body and mind, such as regular exercise, nutritious eating, quality sleep, and stress-reducing practices like meditation or hobbies.

Skincare Rituals: Establish a skincare routine that focuses on nourishing and caring for your skin, promoting its health and radiance.

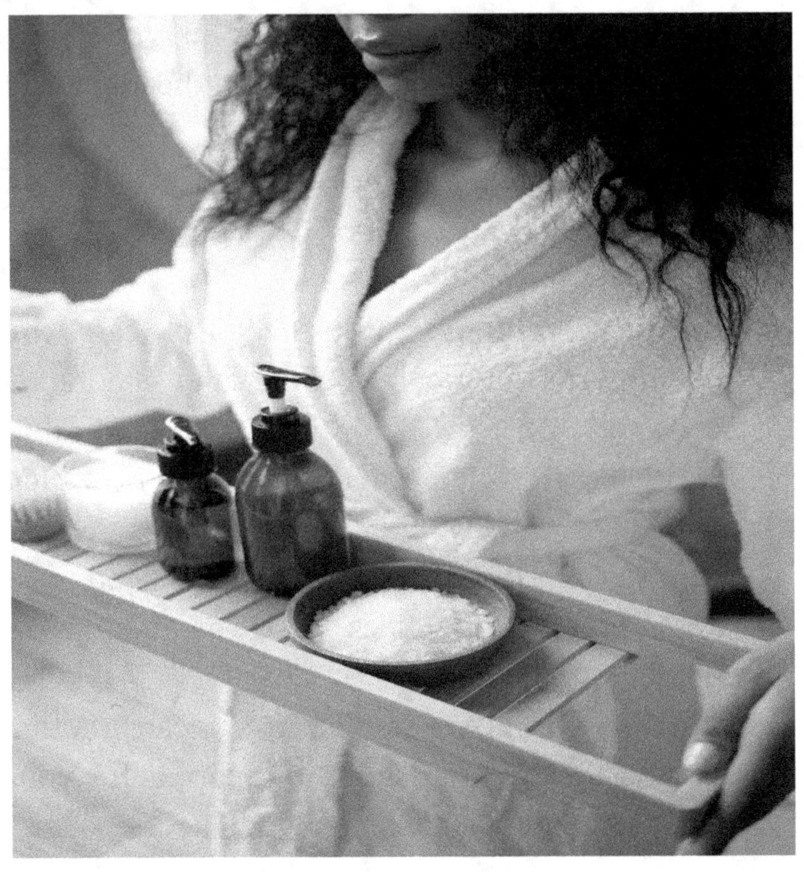

3. **Mindfulness and Gratitude:**

Living in the Present: Practice mindfulness to appreciate the present moment and find joy in everyday experiences, contributing to an inner glow that transcends physical beauty.

Gratitude Practice: Cultivate gratitude for your body's abilities and the journey it has taken you on, fostering a positive self-image.

4. Embracing Individuality:

Authenticity: Celebrate your uniqueness and individuality rather than conforming to societal standards of beauty. Embrace your distinctive features and characteristics.
Confidence: Self-assurance and confidence exude their own form of beauty. Cultivate confidence by recognizing and appreciating your strengths.

5. Continuous Growth and Learning:

Personal Development: Engage in lifelong learning and personal growth. Embrace new experiences, hobbies, or skills that enrich your life, contributing to a more vibrant and fulfilling existence.

Openness to Change: Embrace changes in lifestyle, habits, and perspectives that positively impact your well-being.

6. Cultivating Relationships:

Connection and Support: Foster meaningful connections with others. Building strong relationships and a supportive network can positively influence your mental and emotional well-being, reflecting in your overall beauty.

7. Balance and Moderation:

Well-Rounded Lifestyle: Strive for balance in all aspects of life, including work, leisure, relationships, and self-care.
Healthy Boundaries: Set boundaries to maintain balance and prevent burnout, allowing for sustained well-being.

8. Professional Guidance and Self-Exploration:

Seeking Help When Needed: Consult professionals for advice on skincare, mental health, or any other aspect that impacts your well-being.

Self-Discovery: Explore activities or practices that bring you joy and fulfillment, aiding in a more fulfilled and contented life.

By embracing change gracefully, prioritizing self-care, nurturing a positive mindset, and cultivating a holistic approach to well-being, you can radiate a lasting beauty that transcends the limitations of physical appearance.

Self-care practices for nurturing mental and emotional well-being:

Absolutely, nurturing mental and emotional well-being is crucial for overall health. Self-care practices that focus on mental and emotional wellness can significantly contribute to a healthier mindset and better emotional resilience. Here are some self-care practices for nurturing mental and emotional well-being:

1. **Mindfulness and Meditation:**

Mindfulness Techniques: Practice mindfulness through meditation, deep breathing, or mindfulness exercises to stay present and reduce stress.Mindful Activities: Engage fully in activities like walking, eating, or even showering, focusing on the present moment.

2. **Journaling and Reflection:**

Writing Practice: Maintain a journal to express thoughts, feelings, and reflections. Reflecting on experiences can offer insights and promote self-awareness.Gratitude Journaling: Write down things you're grateful for daily, fostering a positive mindset.

3. **Regular Physical Exercise:**

Mood Enhancement: Exercise releases endorphins, boosting mood and reducing stress.Mind-Body Connection: Practices like yoga or tai chi can help connect the body and mind, promoting relaxation.

4. Quality Sleep:

Sleep Hygiene: Prioritize good sleep habits, aiming for 7-9 hours of quality sleep per night.Bedtime Routine: Establish a calming routine before bed to signal your body it's time to wind down.

5. Setting Boundaries:

Saying No: Learn to say no to commitments that might overwhelm you and set healthy boundaries in relationships.Time Management: Manage time effectively to balance work, personal life, and leisure.

6. Social Connection:

Nurturing Relationships: Spend time with friends, family, or supportive communities to maintain social connections.Open Communication: Share feelings and thoughts with trusted individuals, fostering a sense of belonging and support.

7. **Mindful Nutrition:**

Balanced Diet: Consume a well-rounded diet rich in nutrients that support brain health.Limiting Stimulants: Reduce intake of caffeine and alcohol, which can affect mood and sleep patterns.

8. **Seeking Support:**

Therapy or Counseling: Consider professional help through therapy or counseling to work through challenges and gain new perspectives.Support Groups: Join support groups or communities where you can share experiences and find solidarity.

9. Engaging in Hobbies and Creativity:

Creative Outlets: Pursue hobbies or creative activities that bring joy and fulfillment.Playfulness: Embrace playfulness and laughter as part of your routine.

10. Practicing Self-Compassion:

Self-Kindness: Be gentle with yourself, practicing self-compassion and self-forgiveness.Positive Affirmations: Use positive affirmations to reinforce self-worth and positive self-talk.

By integrating these self-care practices into your routine, you can nurture your mental and emotional well-being, promoting resilience, a positive outlook, and a healthier mindset. Remember, self-care is a personal journey, so find practices that resonate with you and make them a part of your daily life.

Encouraging positive body image and self-acceptance for ageless beauty:

Encouraging positive body image and self-acceptance for ageless beauty involves embracing oneself at every stage of life, valuing inner qualities, and appreciating the beauty that comes with age and experience. Here are some ways to foster positive body image and self-acceptance for ageless beauty:

1. **Embrace Your Unique Self:**

Celebrate Individuality: Embrace your uniqueness, including your body shape, features, and characteristics.Appreciate Changes: Embrace the changes that come with age as a reflection of your life journey and experiences.

2. **Shift the Focus from Appearance:**

Focus on Inner Qualities: Value qualities beyond physical appearance, such as kindness, resilience, wisdom, and compassion.

Holistic Appreciation: Recognize that beauty encompasses mental, emotional, and spiritual aspects, not just physical attributes.

3. Reject Unrealistic Beauty Standards:

Challenge Societal Norms: Advocate for inclusive beauty standards that celebrate diverse ages, body types, and representations in media and society.
Avoid Comparisons: Refrain from comparing yourself to unrealistic or airbrushed images, understanding that true beauty is multifaceted.

4. Practice Self-Compassion:

Positive Self-Talk: Practice positive affirmations and self-encouragement, treating yourself with kindness and understanding.
Self-Forgiveness: Let go of self-criticism and forgive yourself for perceived flaws or imperfections.

5. Nurture Healthy Habits:

Focus on Wellness: Embrace healthy lifestyle choices that promote physical and mental well-being rather than solely focusing on appearance.

Self-Care Practices: Engage in self-care activities that make you feel good and nurtured, fostering a positive relationship with yourself.

6. Cultivate Gratitude and Mindfulness:

Appreciate Your Body: Cultivate gratitude for your body's capabilities, experiences, and the journey it has taken you on.

Mindful Living: Practice mindfulness to appreciate each moment, fostering a more positive and accepting mindset.

7. Surround Yourself with Positivity:

Supportive Environment: Surround yourself with supportive and positive influences, including friends, communities, or social circles that embrace diversity and self-acceptance.

Limit Negative Influences: Minimize exposure to media or environments that perpetuate narrow beauty ideals or negativity.

8. Embrace Aging Gracefully:

Celebrate Life Stages: Embrace the beauty that comes with each stage of life, acknowledging the wisdom and experience gained with age.
Positive Aging: Reframe the narrative around aging, recognizing it as a journey of growth, wisdom, and continued beauty.

9. Educate and Advocate:

Spread Awareness: Educate others about the importance of positive body image and self-acceptance, encouraging inclusivity and diversity.

Advocate for Change: Support movements that challenge ageism and promote body positivity for people of all ages.

Encouraging positive body image and self-acceptance for ageless beauty involves fostering a mindset that appreciates and celebrates oneself beyond societal standards, valuing the inherent beauty found within individuality and life experiences.

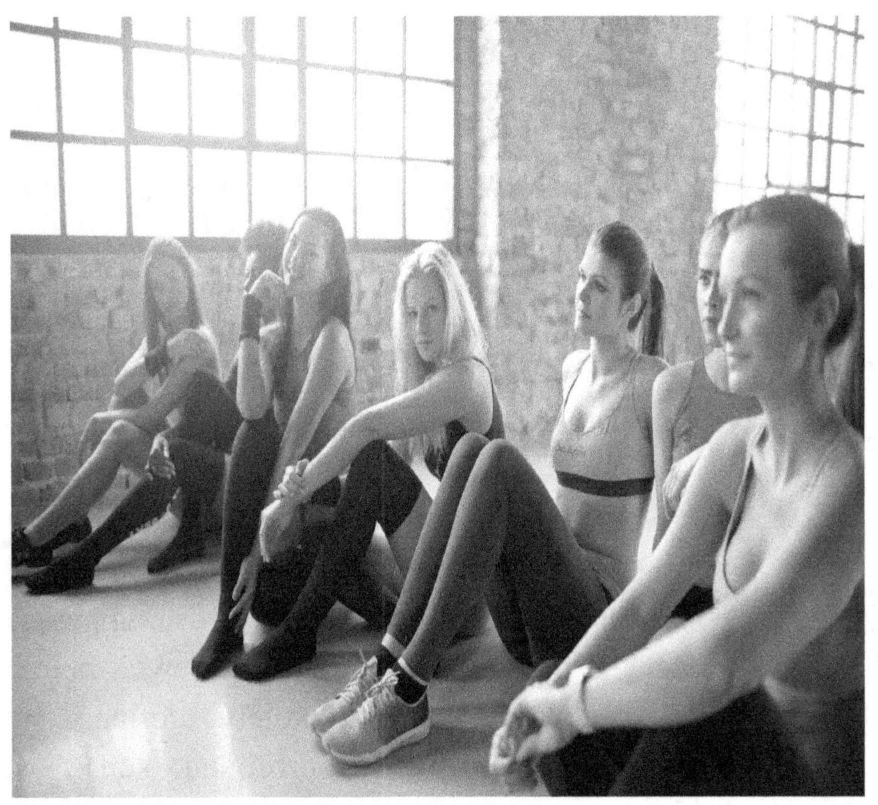

Conclusion

Achieving Ageless Beauty:

In conclusion, achieving ageless beauty transcends conventional perceptions and embraces a holistic approach that encompasses physical, mental, and emotional well-being. Ageless beauty is not solely defined by appearances but by a profound sense of self-acceptance, confidence, and inner radiance that shines through at every stage of life.

Recapitulation of key insights from the book

Whole Well-Being Matters: Beauty isn't just about looks; it's also about feeling good mentally, emotionally, and physically.

Age Is Natural: Embracing aging as a normal part of life helps us feel beautiful at every stage.

Take Care of Yourself: Simple practices like skincare, healthy habits, and managing stress contribute to timeless beauty.

Love Yourself: Self-acceptance and self-love are crucial for feeling beautiful, no matter your age.

Celebrate Diversity: Beauty comes in all shapes, sizes, and ages. Embracing this diversity makes beauty more inclusive.

Stay Positive: Having a positive attitude and confidence shine brighter than any beauty product.

Feel Empowered: Learning, standing up for what you believe in, and feeling confident are all part of being beautifully ageless.

In your pursuit of beauty and well-being, consider embracing a holistic approach that goes beyond skincare routines and delves into nurturing your entire being. True beauty isn't merely skin deep; it's a reflection of your overall health and wellness.

Encouragement to readers to adopt a holistic approach to skincare and wellness

Imagine your skincare routine as a part of a larger, more encompassing picture—one that prioritizes your mental, emotional, and physical wellness. As you embark on this journey, here's some encouragement:

1. **Take Care of Your Mind:** A calm mind emanates beauty, which is more than just outward appearances. Practice mindfulness, meditation, or other techniques to quiet your mind and promote inner peace.

2. **Love Your Body:** Show kindness and respect to your physical form. To promote your skin and general health, adopt a balanced diet, consistent exercise, and enough sleep. Remember that radiant skin is a sign of a healthy body.

3. **Accept Self-Care:** Taking care of yourself is an act of self-love. Enjoy skincare rituals that will both nourish your skin and make you feel better. Make time for things that help you feel refreshed, such as reading, painting, or just going for a leisurely walk.

4. **Seek Balance:** Make it a point to live a balanced life in all felicitations. A happy, stress-free actuality is a result of striking a balance between work, connections, and particular rest. This eventually improves the health of your skin.

5.**Celebrate Individuality:**Your distinct rates and life gusts make you beautiful. Accept and value your tricks and excrescences because they're what truly define your beauty.

6. **Radiate Positivity:** Have an auspicious mindset. Your outlook on life has an impact on your overall good. Accept adversities as chances for development and education

7. **Consistency Is Key:** Just as consistency in skincare routines yields results, consistency in holistic wellness practices bears fruit over time. Make these practices a part of your lifestyle.

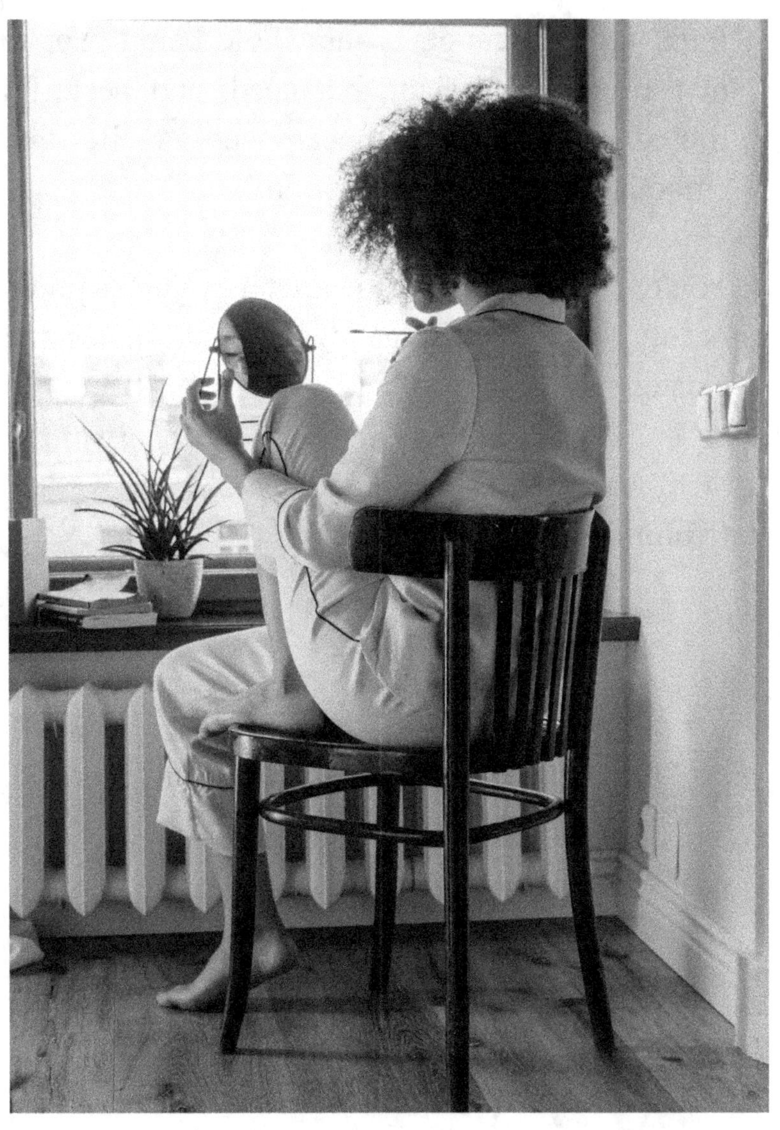

Final thoughts about your whole being. You're investing in a radiant, balanced, and beautiful life that transcends appearances—a life that embodies wellness from within.

You're on a journey towards not just ageless beauty, but a fulfilling, joyous, and wholesome existence.

With warmth and encouragement,
(Mamie C. Fenner)